I0104090

She Learned Her Voice Could Keep Her Safe ~ TJ's Story

ISBN: 979-8-9940500-2-6
Printed in the United States of America
First Edition, 2025

Published by

Sylvain–Davis LightHouse Press™

Sylvain–Davis LightHouse Press™ is the official publisher of this work.
All books, educational materials, and digital resources are produced and distributed under the Sylvain–Davis LightHouse Press™ imprint.

Website: sdlighthousepress.com
Email: sdlighthousepress@gmail.com
Instagram: @sdlighthousepress
Facebook: Sylvain-Davis LightHouse Press

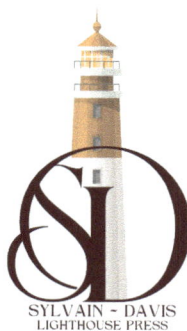

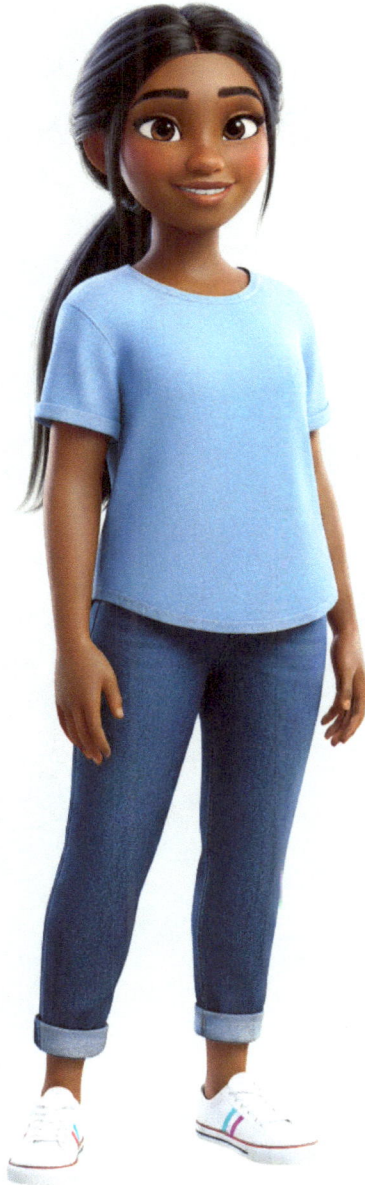

For the children finding their courage, one word at a time.

May you learn, just like TJ, that speaking up is not just brave ~
it can keep you safe.
Your voice is strong, your feelings matter, and you deserve protection.

TJ was good at basketball. Coach Ryan said she had "real talent." He always gave her extra practice time ~ just the two of them.

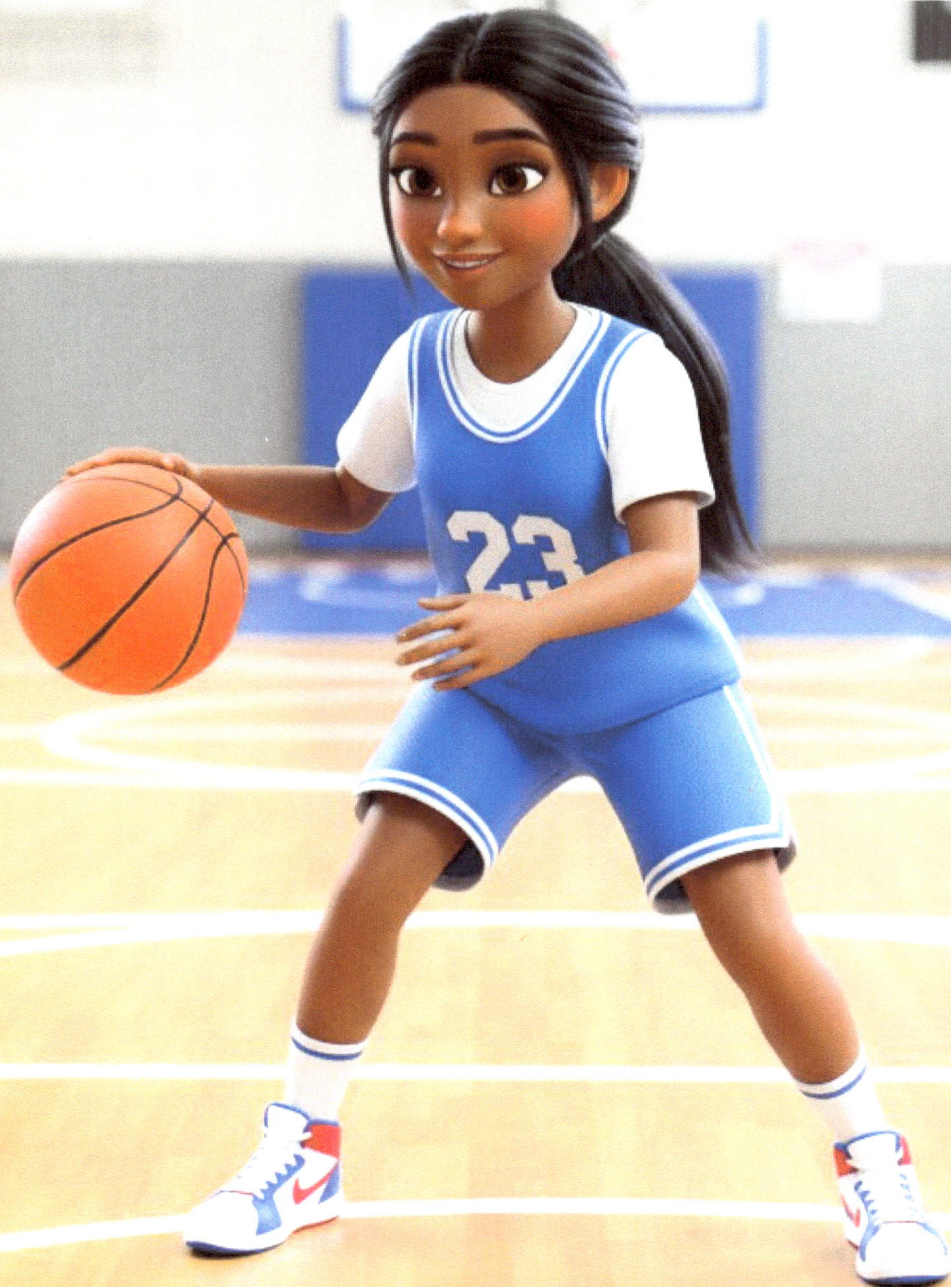

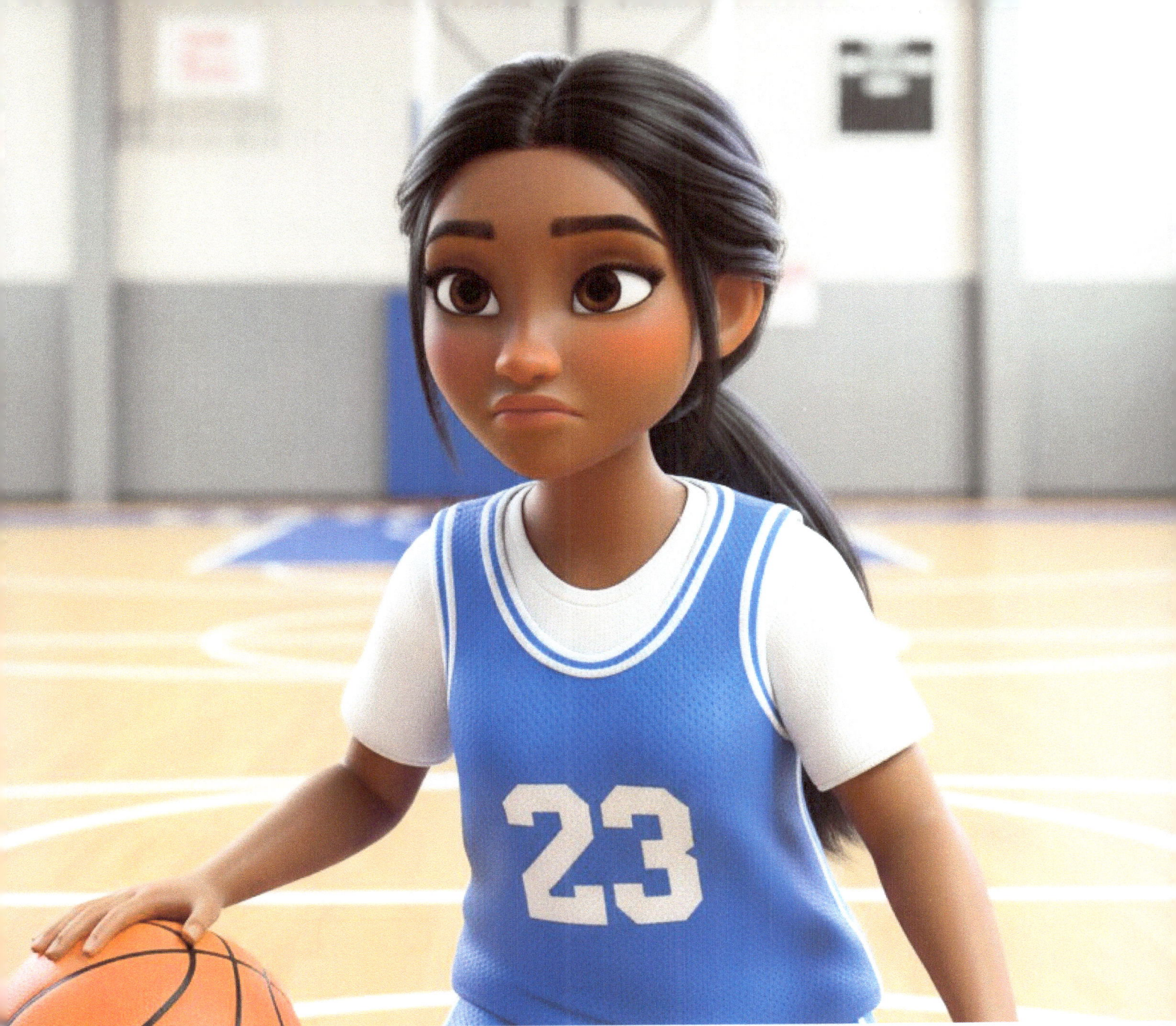

At first, TJ felt proud. But soon, things got...strange.

Coach started giving her gifts ~ a bracelet, new shoes ~ and said, "Don't tell anyone. It's our secret."

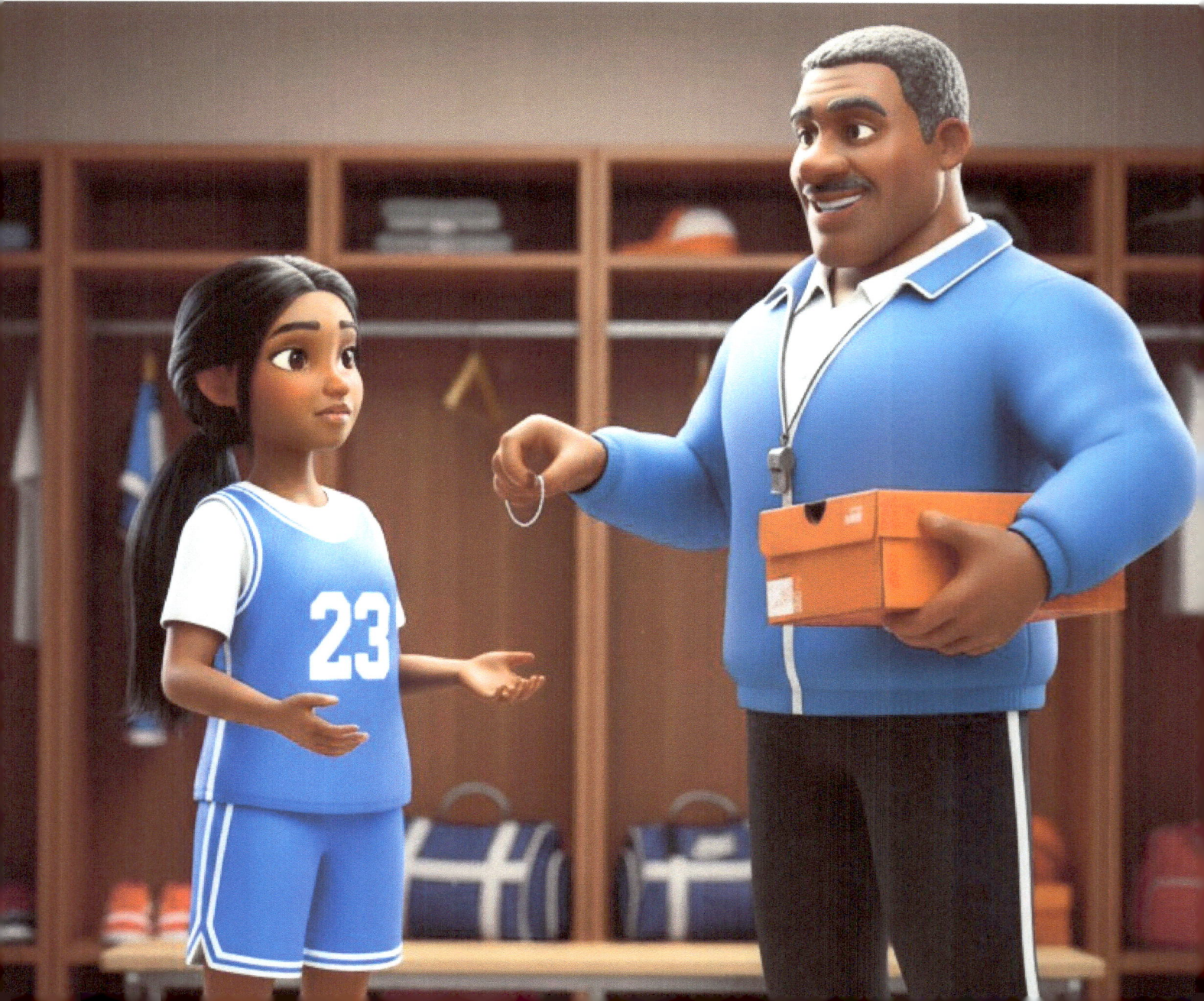

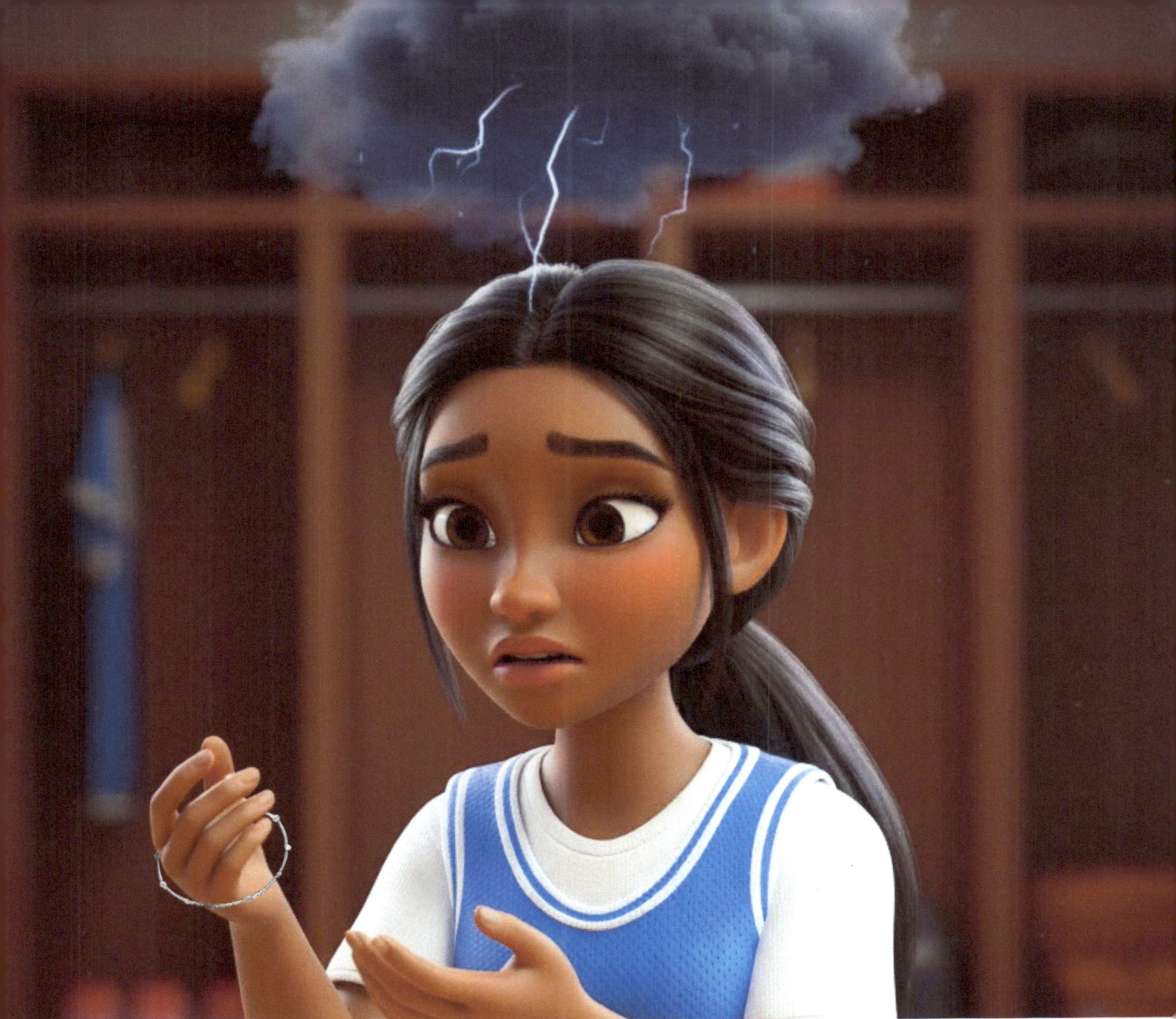

Her stomach tightened. Something didn't feel right.

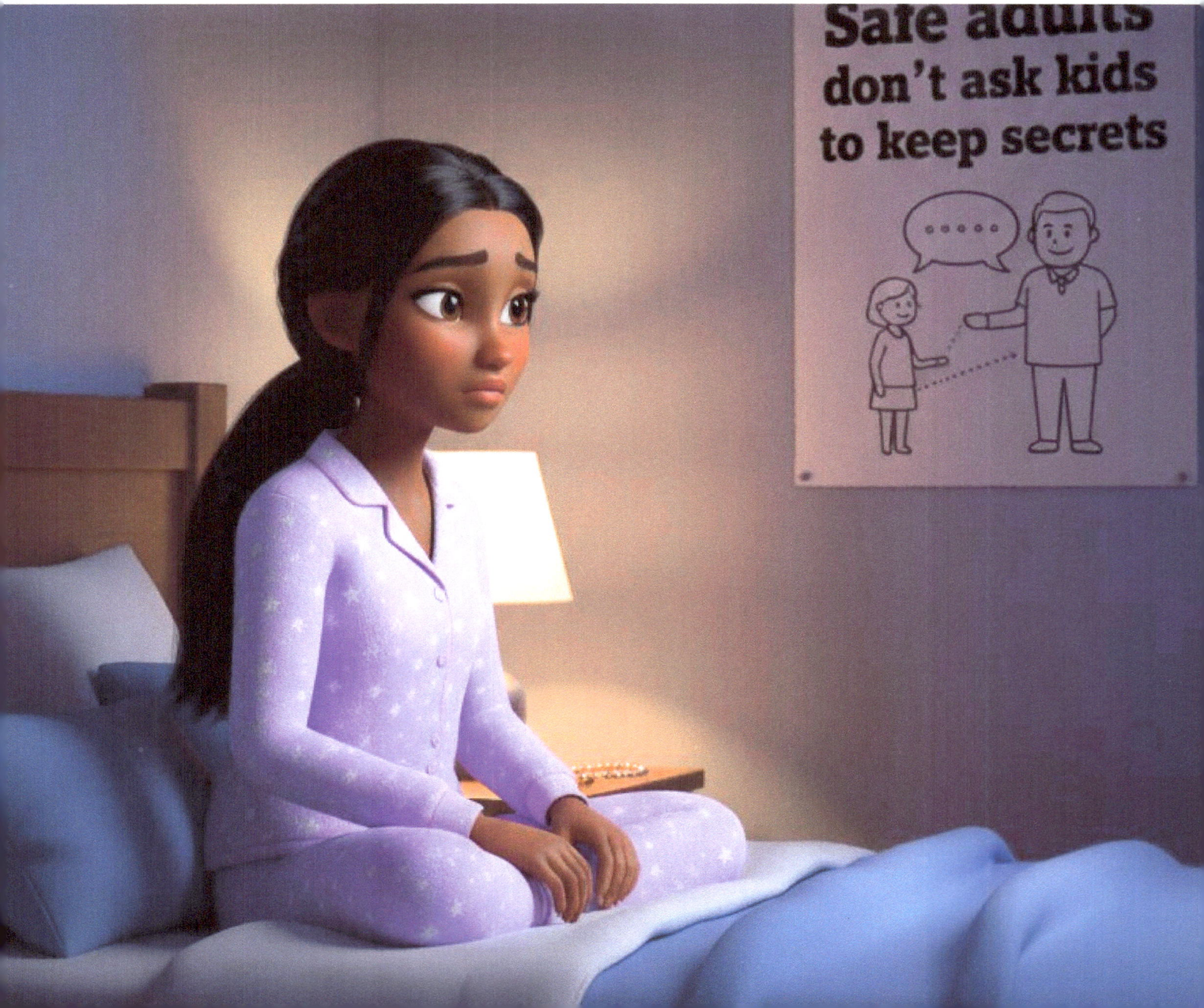

That night, TJ remembered a poster from health class: "Safe adults don't ask kids to keep secrets."

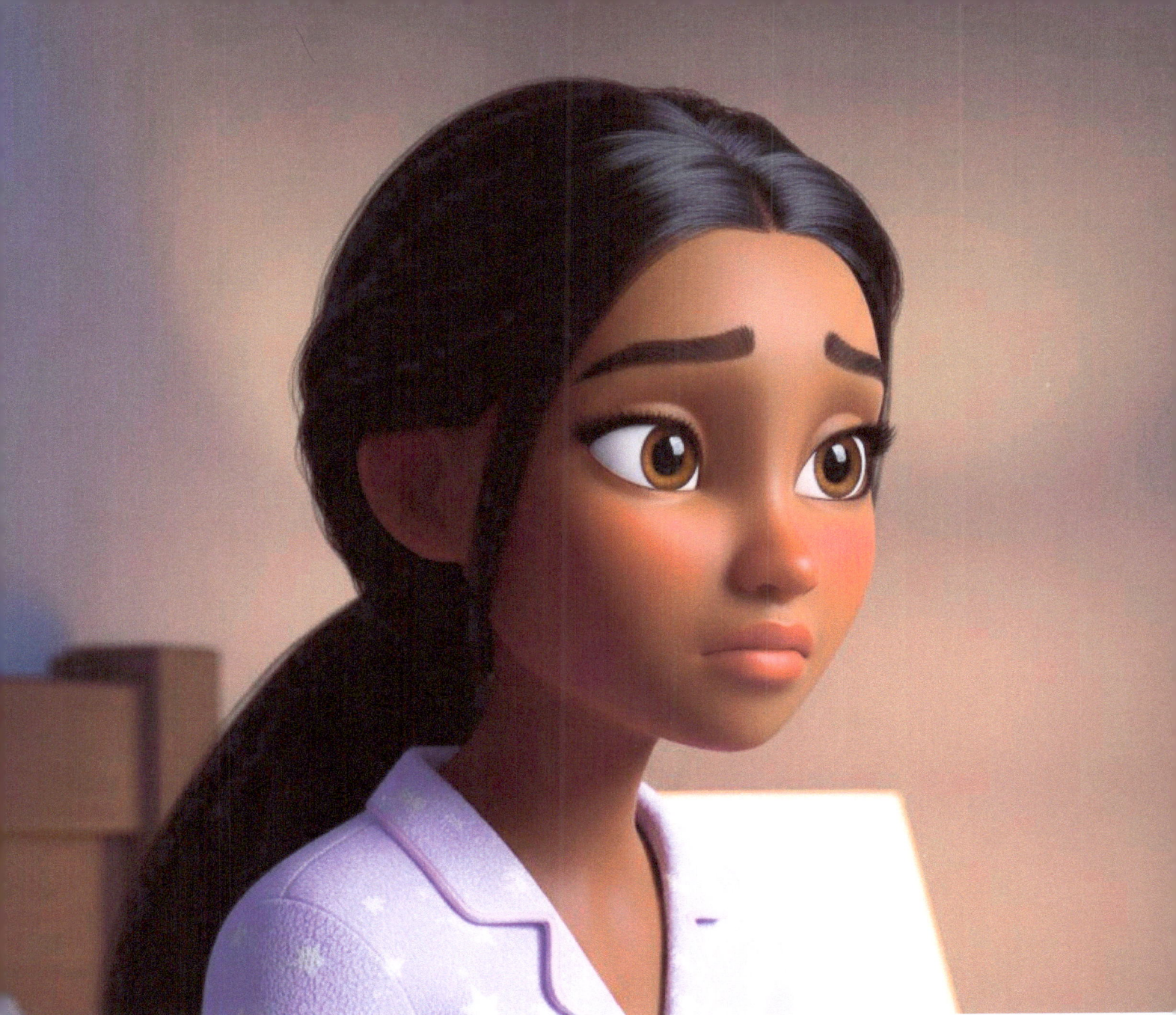

If something feels wrong, it probably is,
she thought.

The next day, she told her friend Kendall,
"I think Coach is crossing a line."

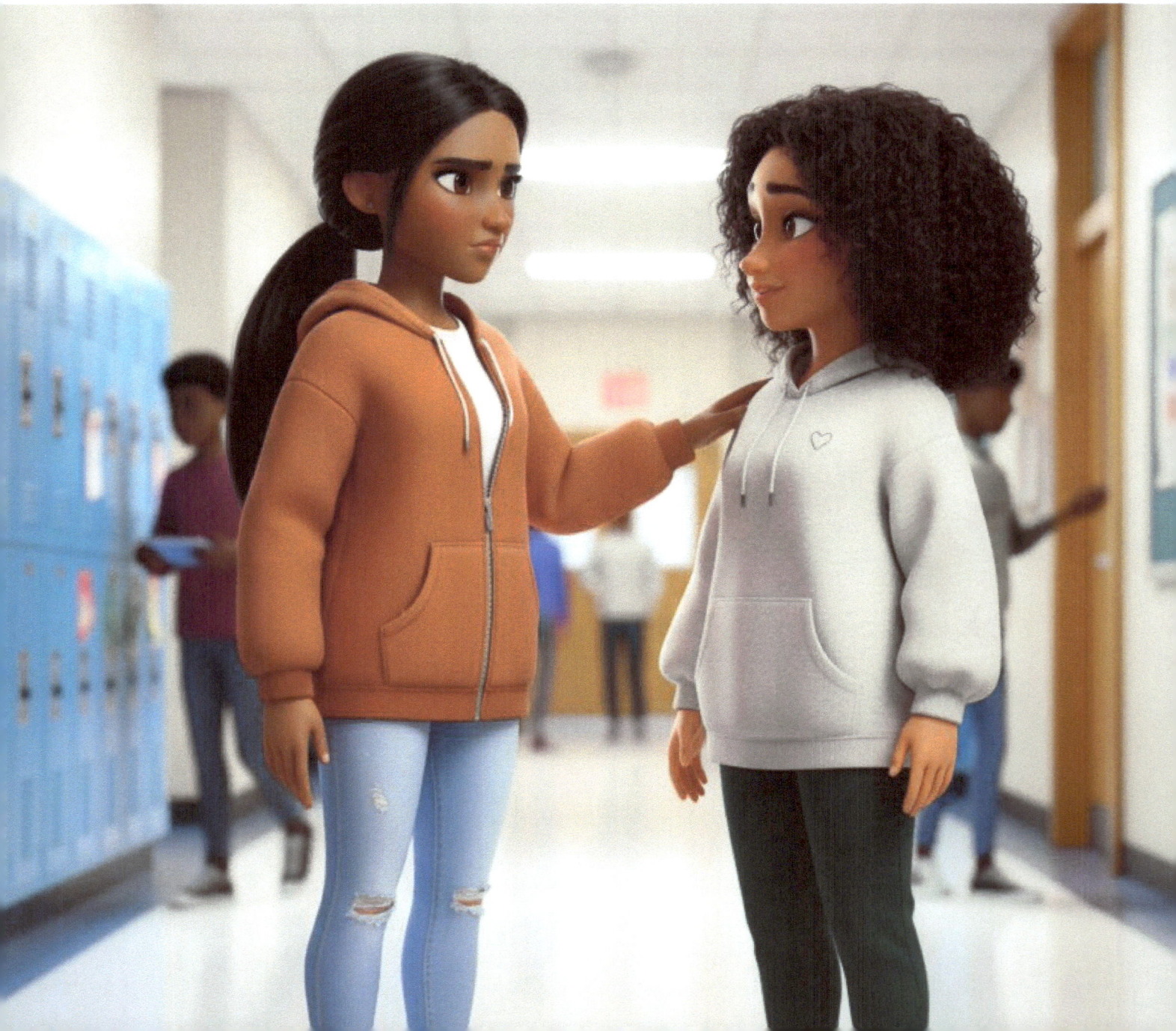

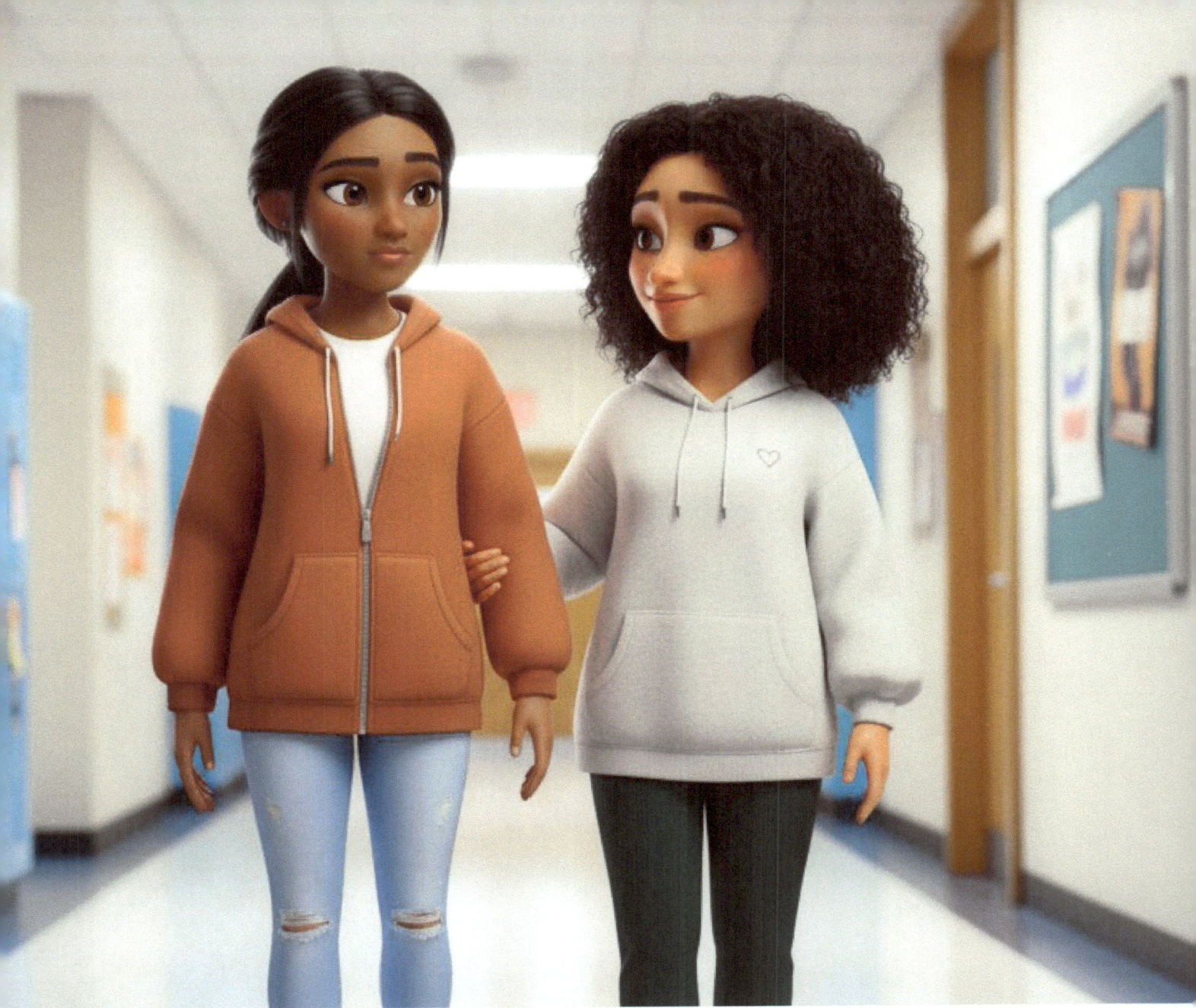

Kendall said, "Let's tell Ms. Bridgett, the counselor.
I'm here for you ~ You're not alone."

Ms. Bridgett listened carefully. "You did the right thing, TJ. You're brave for speaking up."

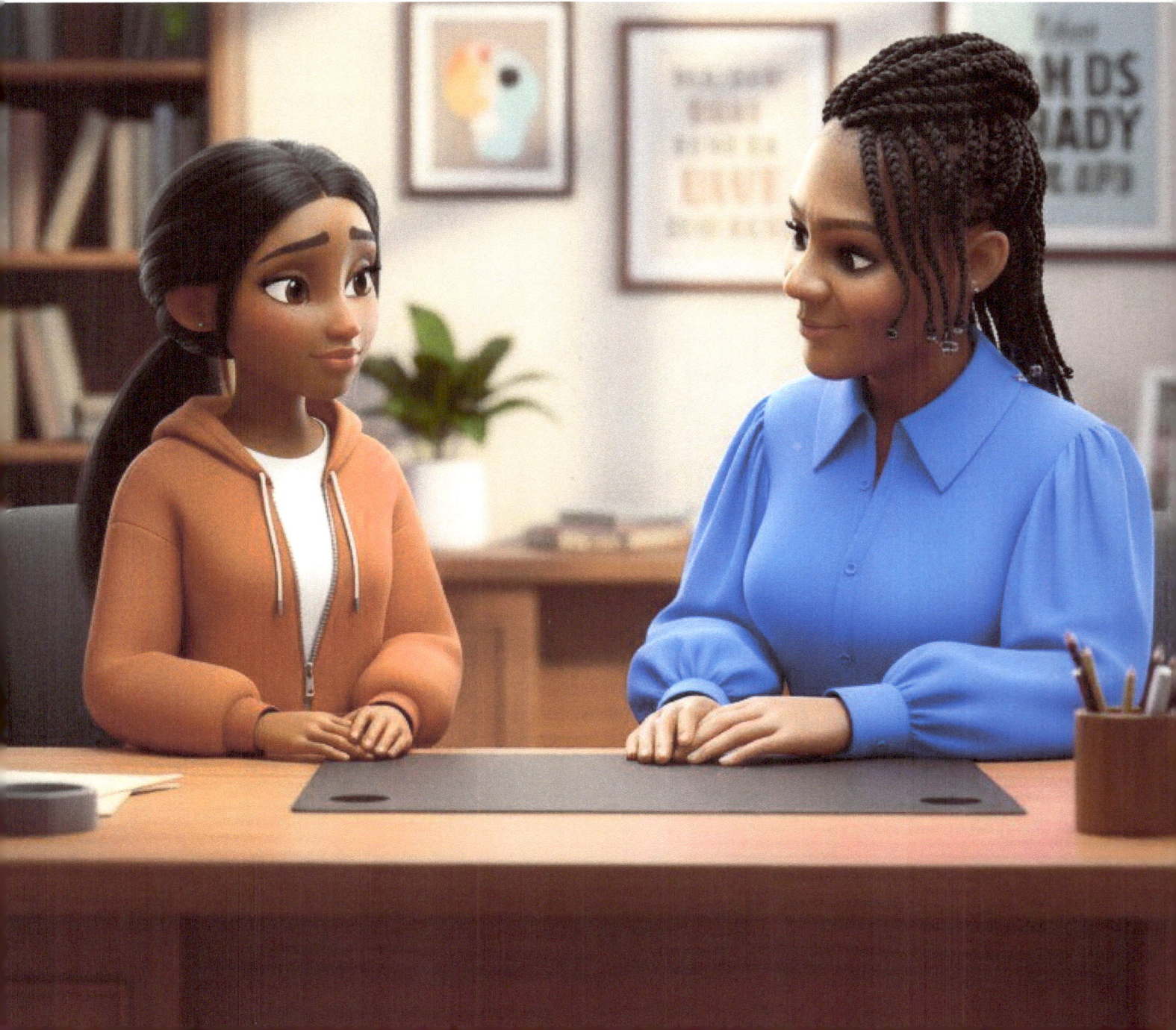

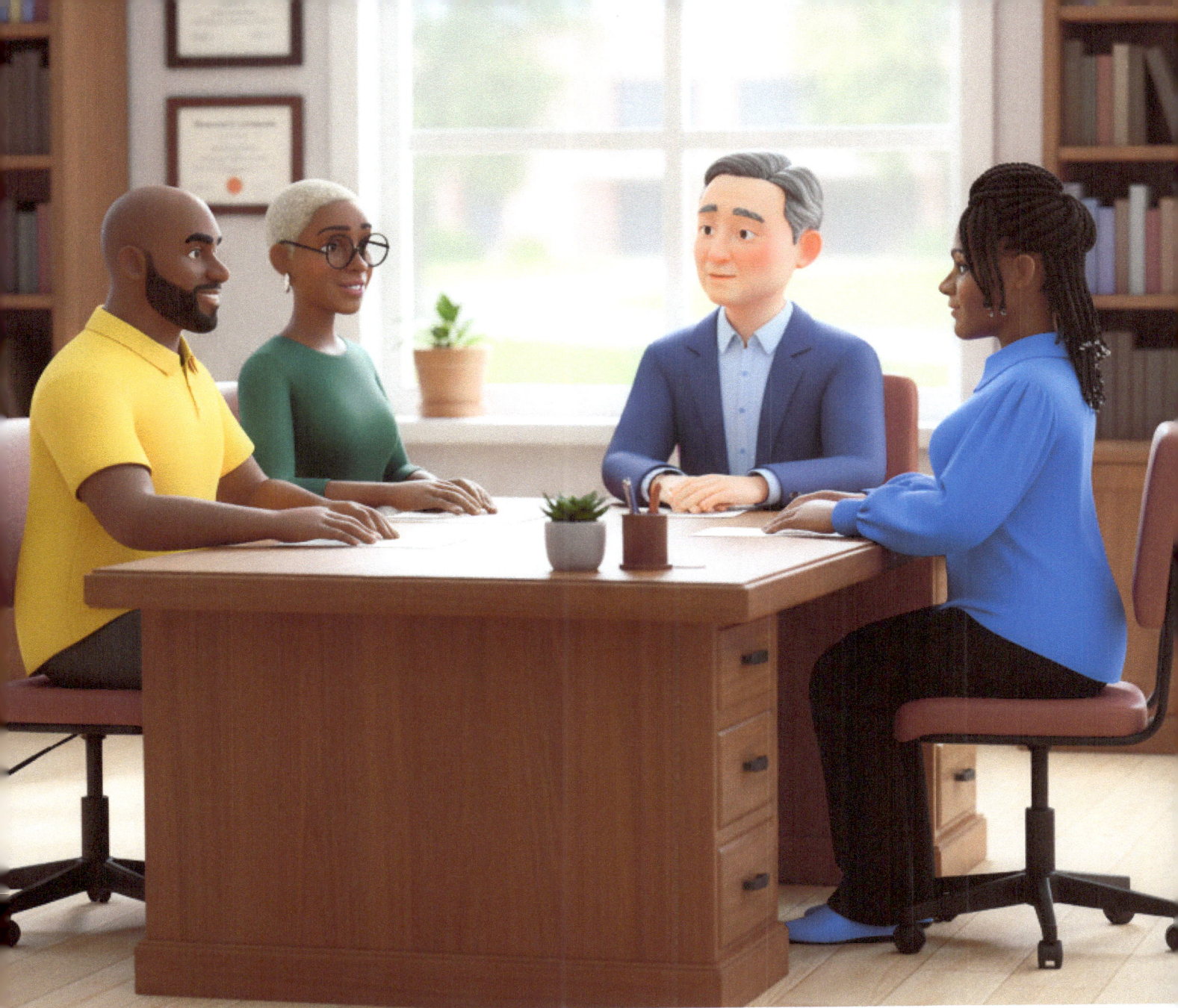

Ms. Bridgett talked to the principal and TJ's parents. They handled it from there.

At the next game, the new coach told the team, "Being strong isn't just about muscles. It's about knowing your boundaries."

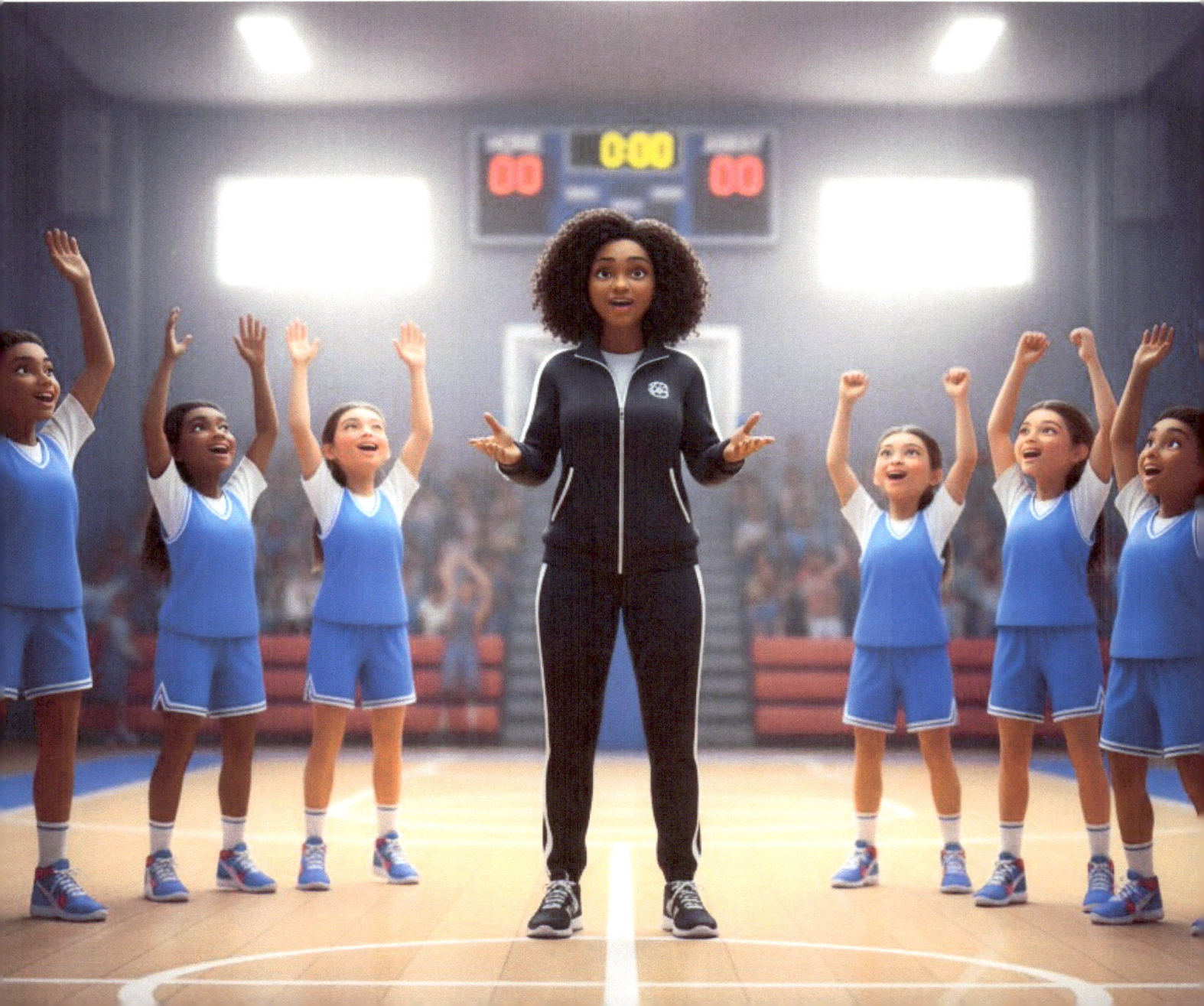

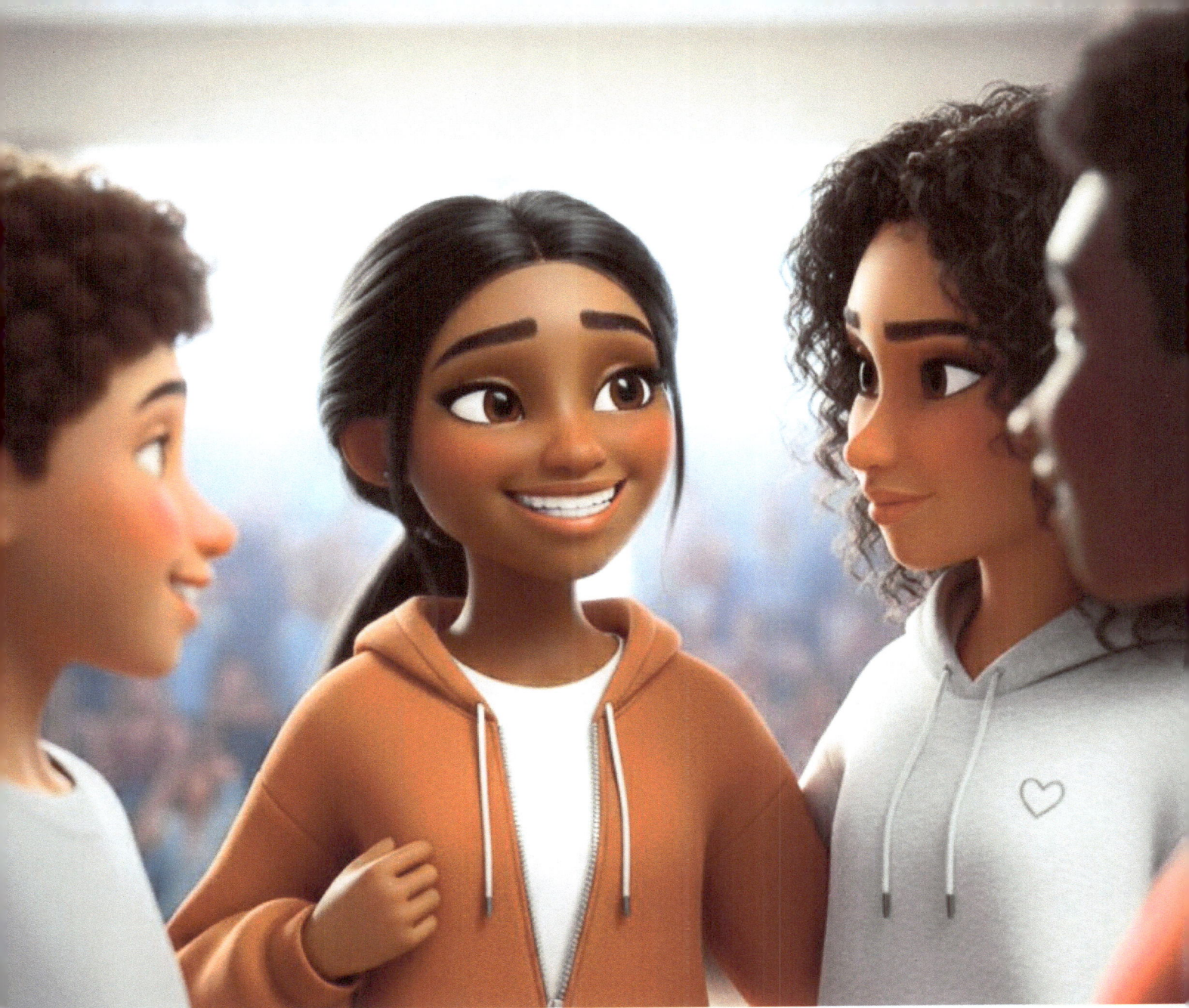

TJ grinned. She learned her voice could keep her safe ~ and her courage could light the way.

TJ's Voice Could Keep Her Safe ~ and Her Courage Could Light the Way

- ☑ I listen to my "uh-oh" feelings.
- ☑ I don't keep secrets that feel wrong.
- ☑ I can say NO and walk away.
- ☑ I tell a trusted adult ~ and keep telling until someone helps.

Parent & Educator Guide

Series: The Child Safety Book Package by Stacy Sylvain-Davis, M.S., M.Ed.
Age Group: Upper Elementary (Ages 8–10)

Learning Objectives:
• Understand healthy vs. unsafe boundaries.
• Recognize signs of grooming or manipulative behavior.
• Encourage assertive communication and self-advocacy.
• Reinforce telling trusted adults when something feels wrong.

Discussion Prompts:
1. What helped TJ realize something wasn't right?
2. How did she find the courage to speak up?
3. Who are the trusted adults in your life?
4. How can we set boundaries with friends, teachers, or online?
5. Why is it important to keep telling until someone helps?

Activities for Children:
• Create a "Trusted Adult Web" - draw circles for the adults you can talk to.
• Journal prompt: "When was a time I used my voice to do the right thing?"
• Practice saying "No" in firm, respectful ways.
• Role-play setting healthy boundaries in digital or school situations.

Tips for Parents & Educators:
• Talk openly about personal boundaries and safe relationships.
• Model assertive but respectful communication.
• Normalize help-seeking behavior - reassure that telling is brave.
• Discuss safe vs. unsafe online interactions.
• Remind children: If something feels wrong, it probably is.

Key Takeaways for Kids:
1. My boundaries deserve respect.
2. My feelings help guide my safety.
3. I can use my voice to say "**No**" and get help.
4. I can always tell a trusted adult and keep telling until someone helps.

Let's Practice Together!

1. What Would You Say?
A grown-up asks you to do something that makes your stomach feel tight or uncomfortable. What can you say?

_____

(Examples: "No, thank you." "I don't like that." "Stop." "I need help.")

2. Safe or Unsafe?
Draw a ✔ next to the safe choices and a ✘ next to the unsafe ones.

☐ A teacher helps you when you fall and scrape your knee
☐ Someone tells you to keep a secret that feels wrong
☐ You ask a trusted adult for help
☐ A grown-up touches you in a way that makes you uncomfortable

3. Who Can I Tell?
Write the names of three safe adults you can go to anytime you feel unsure, scared, or confused.

1. _____
2. _____
3. _____

4. My Brave Words
- **STOP**
- **NO, THANK YOU**
- **I DON'T LIKE THAT**
- **I NEED HELP**
- **THAT MAKES ME UNCOMFORTABLE**

✦ Remember:
Your voice is strong.
Your feelings are important.
And just like TJ, you can always ask for help.

BRAVE & STRONG
CERTIFICATE OF COURAGE

This certificate is proudly presented to:

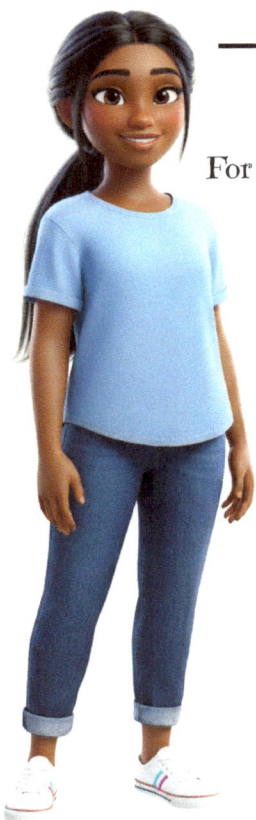

_____

For showing bravery, trusting your feelings, and using your voice ~ just like TJ.
You practiced speaking up, asking for help, and choosing safety.
Your courage makes a difference, and your voice deserves to be heard.

You are strong.

You are important.

You are safe.

You are brave.

Date: _____

Signature: _____

(Parent, Teacher, or Safe Adult)

ABOUT THE AUTHOR

Stacy Sylvain-Davis, M.S., M.Ed., is an educator, author, and advocate dedicated to helping children feel safe, confident, and heard. As a survivor of childhood sexual abuse, she understands the power of a child's voice and the importance of early conversations about safety and boundaries.

With a background in education and years of experience supporting children and families, Stacy creates stories that teach emotional awareness, courage, and self-protection in simple, child-friendly ways.

When she's not writing, she enjoys time with her family and finding joy in life's everyday moments.

ABOUT THE SERIES

The Child Safety Book Package

The *Child Safety Book Collection* is a series of empowering, child-friendly stories designed to help children recognize unsafe situations, trust their feelings, and use their voices with confidence. Through gentle lessons and relatable characters, each book teaches important skills about boundaries, body safety, and speaking up.

Books in the Series:

- **JoJo Says, "No, Thank You!"**
  A story about recognizing unsafe touches and using your voice.

- **Rome and the Secret Box**
  A story about secrets, safe adults, and choosing courage.

- **She Learned Her Voice Could Keep Her Safe: TJ's Story**
  A story about trusting your feelings and asking for help.

This series is designed for families, classrooms, therapists, and ministries who want to protect and empower children with simple, meaningful tools for safety and confidence. Every child deserves to feel safe... and every voice matters.

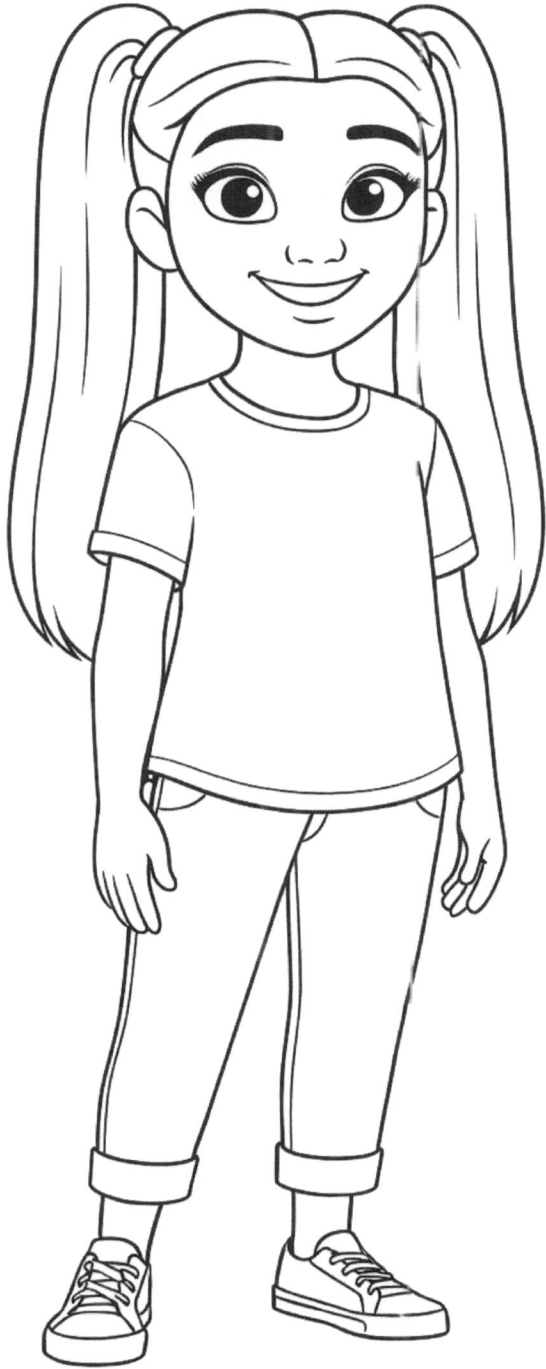

www.ingramcontent.com/pod-product-compliance
Lightning Source LLC
Chambersburg PA
CBHW060828270326
41931CB00002B/101